YOUR KNOWLEDGE HAS VALUE

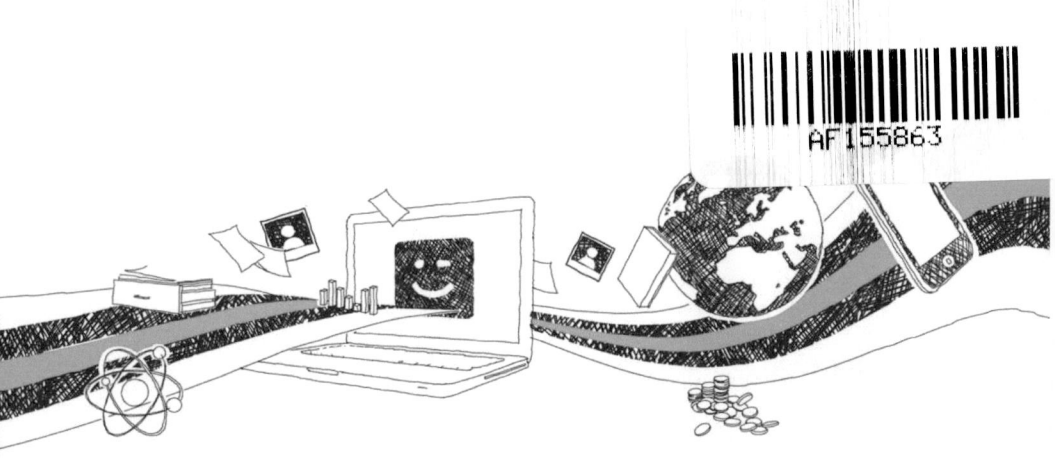

- We will publish your bachelor's and master's thesis, essays and papers

- Your own eBook and book - sold worldwide in all relevant shops

- Earn money with each sale

Upload your text at www.GRIN.com
and publish for free

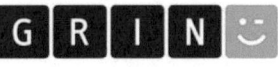

Bibliographic information published by the German National Library:

The German National Library lists this publication in the National Bibliography; detailed bibliographic data are available on the Internet at http://dnb.dnb.de .

This book is copyright material and must not be copied, reproduced, transferred, distributed, leased, licensed or publicly performed or used in any way except as specifically permitted in writing by the publishers, as allowed under the terms and conditions under which it was purchased or as strictly permitted by applicable copyright law. Any unauthorized distribution or use of this text may be a direct infringement of the author s and publisher s rights and those responsible may be liable in law accordingly.

Imprint:

Copyright © 2017 GRIN Verlag, Open Publishing GmbH
Print and binding: Books on Demand GmbH, Norderstedt Germany
ISBN: 9783668470095

This book at GRIN:

http://www.grin.com/en/e-book/359359/antibiotic-regime-of-vascular-pedicled-flap-reconstruction

King Rowis

Antibiotic Regime of Vascular Pedicled Flap Reconstruction

Antibiotic Alternatives In Reconstructive Surgery

GRIN Publishing

GRIN - Your knowledge has value

Since its foundation in 1998, GRIN has specialized in publishing academic texts by students, college teachers and other academics as e-book and printed book. The website www.grin.com is an ideal platform for presenting term papers, final papers, scientific essays, dissertations and specialist books.

Visit us on the internet:

http://www.grin.com/

http://www.facebook.com/grincom

http://www.twitter.com/grin_com

Antibiotic Regime of Vascular Pedicled Flap Reconstruction

Name

Institutional Affiliation

Antibiotic Regime of Vascular Pedicled Flap Reconstruction (1st line and 2nd line therapy regimes)

In order to highlight the problem at hand, intrathoracic defects were chosen to offer an understanding of the key process involved in the reconstruction process. Intrathoracic disorders present numerous distinct challenges and specific issues are related to steady *"dead space"* and bronchopleural fistulae (Ulusal, Liu, & Salgado, 2009). The residual pulmonic section change cannot be in most cases be trusted upon to seal the thoracic *"dead space,"* particularly in *"post-radiotherapy"* cases of clients and this therefore offer a steady setting for empyema and contamination. In this case bronchopleural fistula offers a steady strenuous escape that brands flap devotion particularly hard (Chen, Yazar, Ulusal, Liu, & Salgado, 2009). There are rare core medical standards that try to discourse the issues of *"dead space"* and *"bronchopleural fistula."* The leading standard is associated with the Clagett standard of presented empyema conclusion deprived of straight *"dead space"* destruction and the second is the part of the tissue blinders in bronchial base exposure and lifeless cosmos sealing (Zumla et al., 2010; Chen, Yazar, Ulusal, Liu, & Salgado, 2009). The third one regards to measured conclusion of *"bronchopleural"* fistula by the establishment of a designed air fistula (Chen, Yazar, Ulusal, Liu, & Salgado, 2009). For a description of phased closure of empyema disorders Clagett and Geraci accomplished it by the establishment of a huge exposed opening thoracotomy, and exposed pleural channel debridement (Davies, Davies, & Davies, 2010).

At the time when the strong granulation muscle is existing (although it might take numerous days, the opening is packed with an antibiotic resolution, and the lesion is locked (Zumla et al., 2010). No effort is complete to shut the dead cosmos, even though Clagett`s individual sequence testified about ninety percent overall triumph rate and this has not been simulated by other people even there has been certain potential in a fresh alteration deprived of the usage of exposed thoracostomy (Chen, Yazar, Ulusal, Liu, & Salgado, 2009). It happens in a similar manner just like covering a lesion deprived of the destruction of numb space that seems to display fundamental medical doctrines (Gharagozloo & Cox, 2008).

Moreover, certain scholars have affirmed the necessity for entire sealing with tissue blinders, but this is not a required and not in most cases conceivable (Gharagozloo & Cox, 2008; DuBree & Cox, 2009). Increasingly, an alteration of the Clagett standard can be utilized in combination with tissue blinders, averting the necessity for overall numb space destruction, and hence, the tissue fold is utilized for respiratory treatment instead of capacity substitution (DuBree & Cox, 2009). In accordance, tissue blinders have long been created as a dependable and triumphant strategy for administering intrathoracic reversal of extrathoracic muscle blinders.

Increasingly, free blinkers have been lobbied in disorders where numerous thoracotomies inhibit native tissue reversal. Other people consider the benefits of muscle blinders comprise their part in fighting contagion in investigational and scientific replicas (Zumla et al., 2010). Such offers capabilities imitate to the outlines of a 3D respiratory disorder, re-disclosure of the respiratory base to invulnerable scrutiny, and latent revascularization of ischemic respiratory sections (DuBree & Cox, 2009). Furthermore, Omentum is also illustrated for intrathoracic disorders, nonetheless this possibly link the infected pleural hollow with the *"peritoneum"* besides threats more respiratory concessions from laparotomy and trnsdiaphragmatic transmission (Wang et al., 2011).

Controlled air fistula as a concept is particularly essential in the attendance of bronchopleural fistula, and creation of the *"controlled air fistula"* is achieved by a channel with an inflatable lumen implanted straight into the *"bronchopleural fistula"* (Chen, Yazar, Ulusal, Liu, & Salgado, 2009). It distracts the changing air forces missing from the respiratory base boundaries, permitting the tissue fold progressively flops the channel lumen, shutting the air seepage from the *"controlled air fistula."* Soon afterwards, continuing elimination of the channel over a seven days permits remedial of the succeeding drain path (Chen, Yazar, Ulusal, Liu, & Salgado, 2009). Through diversion of the respiratory fistula in this way, the tissue fold is then offered an enhanced opportunity to the respiratory base.

Literature Review

It is unclear when it comes to describing the precise mastery of fold handling for intrathoracic disorder. It is based on the fact that there are no potential judgments to designate whether initial disorder protection with blinders offers any benefit over prevailing thoracic-surgical preparation " (Chen, Yazar, Ulusal, Liu, & Salgado, 2009; Zumla et al., 2010). Such information occur for intermediate sternotomy disorders, where initial fold protection has been revealed to be greater to debridement and exhaustion, nonetheless it lacks at present-day in intrathoracic disorder (Ulusal, Liu, & Salgado, 2009). In the mainstream of thoracic operating hubs, the plastic specialist is thus engaged merely at a late phase, following botched administration of such disorders (Zumla et al., 2010). The conventional thoracic operating strategy encompasses preliminary *"thoracocentesis"* and beset antibiotic treatment, trailed in the preliminary example by torso conduit location.

Dispute prevails regarding the best strategy following torso duct letdown, with video-aided 'thorascopic' operation 'decortication' and exposed channel with a needful drainage space mutually supported (Zumla et al., 2010). The decortication regards the removal of the recalcitrant gristly coating of the lung that grows in empyema, permitting pulmonic section enlargement. Increasingly, the elimination of numerous ribs (thoracoplasty) to flop the torso fortification rests a twilight alternative in various situations (Zumla et al., 2010). Nevertheless it is not the solution that might be anticipated, with letdown proportions of an average of twenty-five percent significant enhancing deformity, and unfavorable impacts such as empyema, nonetheless nothing as however prevails that encompass the initial part of fold protection (Zumla et al., 2010).

Empyema and Pedicled Flap Alternatives Conserved

The usage of a fold rebuilding for optimal results is mandated by the incidence of a 'bronchopleural fistula.' The Clagett process employed in these instances has been traditionally linked with an elevated letdown rate (DuBree & Cox, 2009). Regional flaps that comprise of latissimuss dorsi can be rearranged into the torso to conceal the respiratory base. There are various essential aspects concerning the triumphant administration of the disorders, except merely rearranging tissue (Brandt & Alvarez, 2012). The tissue fold at first is not majorly sewed to the friable respiratory muscles, however is merely swathed over them. It associates with the next idea in which remedial of the respiratory fistula tissue fold boundary is thus attained by spineless and rigid gauze stuffing and the usage of a calculated air fistula (DuBree & Cox, 2009). The usage of a *"designed air fistula"* marks the third pointy and it employs an even silicone drain (10mm) that permits alterations in pressure (Ulusal, Liu, & Salgado, 2009). In so doing, it helps to bypass the respiratory base-tissue flap boundary and hence enable the devotion of the tissue fold to respiratory base limits.

The lumen of the channel can be destroyed by force employed by rigid gauze filling. Hence, the *"designed air fistula"* can be locked a few days following a preliminary operation, when respiratory tissue fold lesion remedial is well in progress (Brandt & Alvarez, 2012). The channel is steadily detached over a few days to permit remedial of the channel path. The other thing is that as a solitary pedicled flap hardly offers enough capacity to destroy numb cosmos, the Clagett standard is utilized in combination with the Pedicled flap to permit dead space conclusion (DuBree & Cox, 2009). Once lenient and rigid gauze filling has been completed, and the *"designed air fistula"* has been detached, the quantity of gauze stuffing is steadily diminished over the subsequent days. Moreover, conclusive destruction of numb cosmos emanates from 'mediastinal' and 'diaphragmatic' change.

Increasingly, when provincial blinders have been separated by preceding thoracotomies (this might comprise of manifold botched 'decortication' and exposed 'bronchopleural' fistula overhaul efforts) and free blinders can be utilized (Chen, Yazar, Ulusal, Liu, & Salgado, 2009; DuBree & Cox, 2009). They are characteristically extracted from the 'contralateral' torso barricade, even though the use of the thigh is epithelialized has been described. Notwithstanding the statistic that superior capacities can be attained with free blinders, it is realized that in 'post-pneumonectomy' instances, the Clagett standard has in most cases been utilized to shut numb space (Schneiter, Grodzki, & Lardinois et al., 2008). It ought to be realized that even when the confined tissues have been separated by preliminary 'thoracotomies.' The residual 'proximal' shares are still important for safeguarding of micro vascular 'anastomoses' and for increasing of the lenient muscle capacity introduced into the thoracic hollow.

Evidence Review and Procedure for Treatment

Proof for the operation handling of 'intrathoracic' disorders that comprises of "bronchopleural fistula" besides empyema is not available (Zumla et al., 2010). There are no potential judgments relating thoracic as well as plastic operating strategies to such disorders with the mainstream of plastic medical involvements having been presented in reflective instances sequences (Ulusal, Liu, & Salgado, 2009). Even though there are certain proof associating diverse sorts of thoracic medical involvements, it does not benefit people respond to some basic inquiries (Schneiter, Grodzki, & Lardinois et al., 2008; Zumla et al., 2010). It is so since there no clarity regarding the phase in which a flap reconstruction ought to be regarded and it is also not clear if flap makeover is grander to a thoracic medical process. Until the time when such inquiries will be responded to the two strategies to handling intrathoracic disorders ought to be regarded harmonizing as opposed to being reciprocally select(Brandt & Alvarez, 2012). Nonetheless, an idea ordinarily recognized by individually thoracic and plastic doctors is that the "bronchopleural fistula" ought to be shut with whichever loco regional or unrestricted blinders so that the empyema cosmos can be shut (Zumla et al., 2010).

Given the unavailability of proof concerning optimal management of intrathoracic disorders, a procedure for treatment cannot be viewed as conclusive (Lee & Lawrence, 2010).

When modest procedures like torso conduit channel have not succeeded, it is unclear if thoracic medical involvements or a fold process ought to be the subsequent preferable phase (Brandt & Alvarez, 2012). There is a disagreement regarding the previous usage of tissue flap restoration instead of conventional Clagett process in chosen clients (Zumla et al., 2010). Hence, it is based on its comparatively meager accomplishment that has been recorded as squat as twenty percent and the prolonged management sequence that is in typical terms six months from exposed "thoracostomy" to lesion closure (Lee & Lawrence, 2010; Ulusal, Liu, & Salgado, 2009). The relational triumph proportions of tissue flap processes are elevated at about eighty-eight percent than conventional Clagett process, with unkind hospital visits of close to thirty days for tissue flap processes (Brandt & Alvarez, 2012). Nonetheless, there is continued lobby for the utilization of the Clagett process as 1st-line management in secluded empyema as in other clusters (Brandt & Alvarez, 2012). It ought to be celebrated that there is potential in a recent alteration of the Clagett process deprived of exposed "thoracostomy" with triumph proportions up to a hundred percent. When the Clagett process is employed, it is suggested that usage of the alteration presented by Gharagozloo et al. It people anticipate to witness if preliminary tissue flap restoration is grander to the Clagett process as 1st-line management in 'intrathoracic' disorders and this is an extent that imposes extra examination (Brandt & Alvarez, 2012).

Here, the strategy regards two important aspects that comprise of the incidence of 'bronchopleural fistula' then is considered to mandate a medical fold termination for the huge opportunity of triumph (Schneiter, Grodzki, & Lardinois et al., 2008). It is precisely in post-radiotherapy patients with imperfect capability for post-operative destruction by the increase (Schneiter, Grodzki, & Lardinois et al., 2008; Brandt & Alvarez, 2012). The conventional Clagett process is not precisely triumphant in the incidence of *"bronchopleural fistula,"* as the bulk of letdowns in the main sequences were featured in the incidence of *"bronchopleural fistula"* (Zumla et al., 2010). It is then clear that Clagett process is not appropriate as 1st-line management in the incidence of *"bronchopleural fistula"* (Brandt & Alvarez, 2012). The 'comorbid' besides nourishing position of the client impacts the situation regarding if the client has a solitary phase or multiphase fold process (Ulusal, Liu, & Salgado, 2009). In cases where the client is not improved for operation, it is recommended that a staged strategy is used with the main flap process reserved following a preliminary effort at 'endoscopic' 'bronchopleural fistula' shutting, exposed channel, and antagonistic nutritive contribution (Lois & Noppen, 2011). There is developing proof for 'endoscopic' treatment of trivial 'bronchopleural fistula' besides this is forecast to be one of the utmost alterations in the prospect of treating intrathoracic disorders (Lois & Noppen, 2011).

Free Flaps versus Pedicled Flaps

The utmost sequence of Pedicled flaps in intrathoracic disorders comprise of a hundred incidences in relationship with sequences of unrestricted blinders for which the utmost had seven circumstances. It is thus, hard to lure authentic deductions concerning their comparative advantages (Lois & Noppen, 2011). The inclusive triumph proportions are identical with Pedicled blinders pronounced at more than seventy percent and free flaps at about ninety-two percent. The key benefit in relation to results seem to be in the treatment of 'bronchopleural fistula,' probably based on the capacity to change the fold to the disorder, the obtainability of grander muscle substance and enhanced "*vascularity*" (Lee & Lawrence, 2010) Pedicled blinders have a recorded triumph frequency of more than sixty percent in relation to that of free flaps that stands at about ninety percent (Lois & Noppen, 2011).

Increasingly, the comparative advantages of unrestricted and pedicled blinders although there are particular clients in whom the usage of pedicled blinders is unbearable, when it is based on manifold thoracotomies, insufficient reach or bulk or preceding letdowns (Lois & Noppen, 2011). There are numerous case sequences recording excellent triumph proportions with beyond twenty four cases recorded in the literature (Lois & Noppen, 2011). The "*rectus abdominus*" besides the latissimuss dorsi are the record shared free blinders employed in 'intrathoracic' disorders in these sequences however they portray numerous disadvantages. Such comprise of side placing for reaping the latissimuss dorsi flap that need patient relocation and creating a double squad strategy unbearable (Ulusal, Liu, & Salgado, 2009). Stomach cuts for reaping of "*rectus abdominus*" or 'omentum' might impact previously negotiated thigh musculocutaneaus flap that permits a two team strategy, plentiful tissue capacity, and negligible contributor location indisposition (Wang et al., 2011; Lois & Noppen, 2011).

It is important to note that, intrathoracic disorders remain a puzzling issue for the reconstructive specialist with meager patient composition and an elevated indisposition notwithstanding medical involvement indisposition (Wang et al., 2011). The usage of unrestricted or pedicled tissue blinders in combination with the philosophies of the Clagett process and the conception of the "*designed air fistula*," permit a supplementary measured and productive shutting of such disorder (Lois & Noppen, 2011; Lee & Lawrence, 2010). Triumph proportions that near a hundred percent are possible utilizing such strategies. Nonetheless, there is presently little superior information on the optimum management for 'intrathoracic' disorders and on if reconstructive specialists ought to be engaged at an formerly phase as opposed to following manifold failed decortication and drainage processes indisposition (Wang et al., 2011).

References

Brandt, C., & Alvarez, J. M. (2012). "First-line treatment of deep sternal infection by a plastic surgical approach: superior results compared with conventional cardiac surgical orthodoxy." *Plast Reconstr Surg*. 2231-2237.

Chen, H. C., Yazar, S., Ulusal, A. E., Liu, Y. T., & Salgado, C. J. (2009). "Tissue plug technique for management of large chronic empyema defects and bronchopleural fistulas." *J Reconstr Microsurg*. 25:213-218.

Davies, H. E., Davies, R. J., & Davies, C. W. (2010). "BTS Pleural Disease Guideline Group. Management of pleural infection in adults: British Thoracic Society Pleural Disease Guideline 2010." *Thorox*. 65(2): 41-53.

DuBree, K. J. & Cox, J. L. (2009). "Pleural space irrigation and modified Clagett procedure for the treatment of early postpneumonectomy empyema." *J Thorac Cardiovasc Surg*. 116:943-948.

Gharagozloo, F., & Cox, J. L. (2008). "Pleural space irrigation and modified Clagett procedure for the treatment of early postpneumonectomy empyema." *J Thorac Cardiovasc Surg*. 116:943-948.

Lee, S. F., & Lawrence, D. (2010). "Thoracic empyema: current opinions in medical and surgical management." *Curr Opin Pulm Med*. 16:194-200.

Lois, M., & Noppen, M. (2011). "Bronchopleural fistulas: an overview of the problem with special focus on endoscopic management." *Chest*. 128:3955-3965.

Schneiter, D., Grodzki, T., & Lardinois, D., et al. (2008). "Accelerated treatment of postpneumonectomy empyema: a binational long-term study." *J Thorac Cardiovasc Surg*. 136:179-185.

Wang, T., et al. (2011). "One-stage pedicled omentum majus transplantation into thoracic cavity for treatment of chronic persistent empyema with or without bronchopleural fistula." *Eur J Cardiothorac Surg*. 636-638.

Zumla, A. et al. (2010). "Thoracic empyema: current opinions in medical and surgical management." *Curr Opin Pulm Med*. 16:194-200.

YOUR KNOWLEDGE HAS VALUE

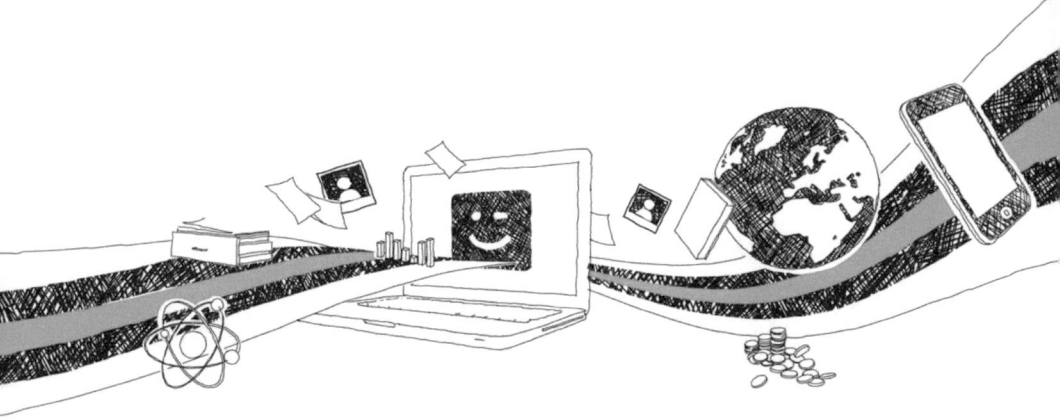

- We will publish your bachelor's and master's thesis, essays and papers

- Your own eBook and book - sold worldwide in all relevant shops

- Earn money with each sale

Upload your text at www.GRIN.com and publish for free

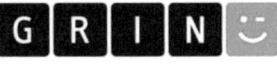